Essential Oils Guide:

30 Amazing Summer Refreshing Blends for Your Home

Table of content:

Introduction: Is your home summer ready?

Do you know how to use essential oils to calm the anxious, increase mental focus, and help your concentration? Do you want your home to be healthy, happy, and toxin-free while introducing aromas to help your home feel like summer on the inside? This book is done for that one purpose. It will walk you through everything you need to know on how to mix your own essential oil blends for the diffuser. This book will explain what to expect from each of the essential oils. I will even give you advice on how to use essential oils when you do not have or can't afford your own diffuser. So, if you're ready to take charge of freshening your home without spending money on synthetic fragrances, you need to buy this book.

Chapter 1 - What is Aromatherapy?

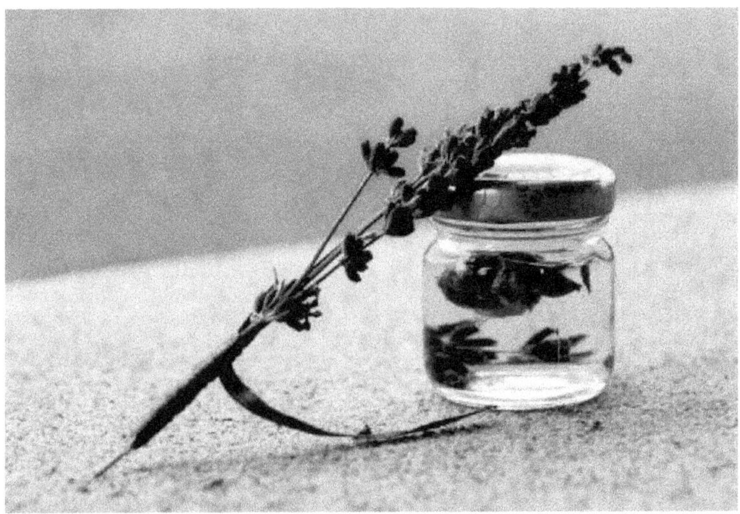

Fragrant plants and the oils from those plants have been used for thousands of years for incense, perfume, colognes, and cosmetics. They have also been used for ritual purposes and cleansing rituals. Ancient Egyptians used essential oils in their embalming practices. There is even historical evidence stating they were used for medicinal purposes.

Essential oils are the most concentrated form of the plant. It is made by distilling the plant and collecting the oil, placing it in a bottle. It is then put in blends with other essential oils for a myriad of different uses. It works by activating the limbic system of the brain which can stimulate nerve receptors to promote calming, healing, and even help boost the immune system.

There are many tools you can use to make essential oil products, but in order to have the fragrance float through the air, you will need a diffuser, or something you can use as one. You can use essential oils undiluted in the diffusers since they will not come in contact with your skin.

There is more than one type of diffuser you can use.

Plug-in

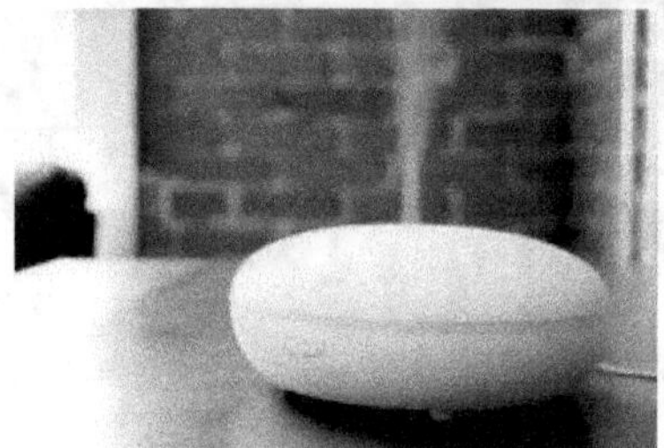

This is the main type of diffuser. As its name states, it gently warms the essential oils by using electricity. They come in different size and can be very pricey, depending on brand.

Reed Diffuser

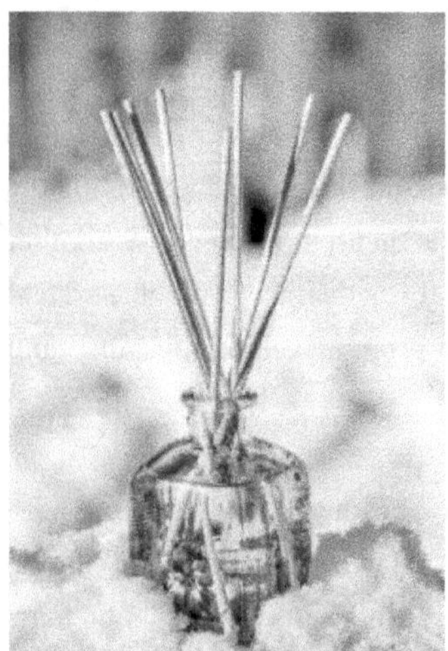

You can find these in any department or super store. They are one of the cheaper alternatives. It is used by placing the oils in the bottle and then placing the reeds in the oil. Due to the capillary nature of the bamboo reeds, the essential oil is naturally draw up the reed and dispersed. No heat is required.

There are two disadvantages:

1.   The only disadvantage is the fragrance not being very prevalent throughout the home.

2. You will have to scrub out the bottle if you do not rinse it between uses.

Potpourri Burner

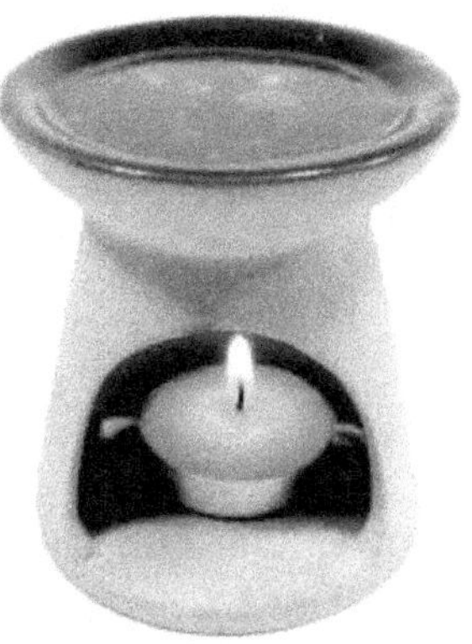

These are as easy to find as the ones above. All you do is place the oil blend in the top and light a candle. As the clay heats up, the essential oils are activated, releasing the aroma into the air.

There are some things around the house you can use to diffuse the essential oils into the air in your home.

Candle warmer

You can use a candle warmer as a diffuser by placing ten drops of essential oils on the warming plate and turning it on.

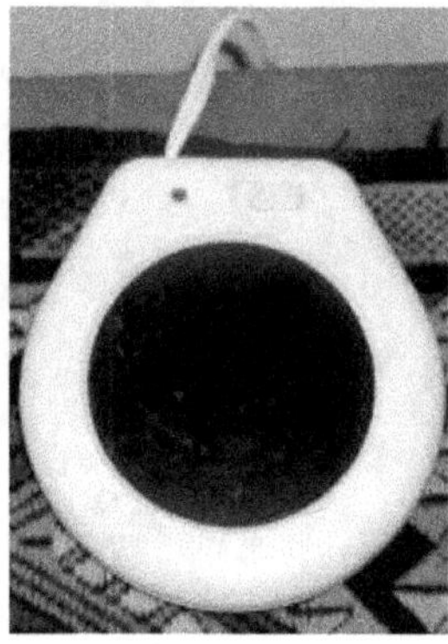

Light Bulb

This is a last resort substitute, but it does work in a pinch. Place up to four drops of an essential oil or blend on the top of the bulb before you turn on the light. **Do not place the essential oils on hot bulb.** Essential oils are flammable. They have to be heated slowly in order for them not to ignite.

You can also place the essential oils on a small plate in the sun to activate them and disperse the aroma through the air. The sun will be enough to heat the oils as long as they are in direct sunlight.

Chapter 2 - Calming the Mood

Between bills, work, family, and running errands, you have one thing in common with a lot of other people, stress. It make you irritable, lose sleep, and even create anxiety. Stress can also manifest as physical diseases.

Coping with stress

In our lives, we try to cope with stress and often find we fall short in doing so. We want to be able to handle everything that is thrown our way only to find that we are in over our heads. Here are a few things you can try to help you cope with everyday stress.

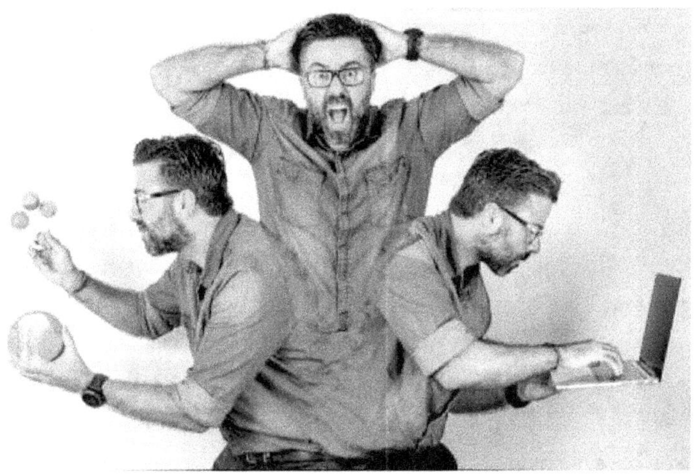

1. Unplug

This may be the hardest thing to do in today's world of computers, laptops, and tablets, not to mention smart phones. Make it a point to step away from the internet and turn off your phone.

You can listen to music to help you relax as long as you are not on the internet, on the phone, or texting. Your mind needs to relax, too. It can't do this with all the stimuli you have around you and all the information you are constantly inputting into your mind.

2. Spoil yourself

If unplugging is the hardest, the second hardest is to be selfish. Yes, you have to spoil yourself every once in a while. Do what you want to do and what makes you happy, and you have to do it every day. This will help relieve stress.

3. Take up a hobby that isn't electronic

This can be reading a physical book, drawing, crochet, or any other hobby that doesn't require you to turn on a computer or tablet. Why? When you actively practice your hobby, your has the habit of putting all the daily stresses to the back of your mind to focus on what you are doing in that moment. This relieves stress.

4. Meditation

This is the act of clearing your mind and focusing on nothing but your breathing. You can use this technique to relax muscles, relieve stress and even help you sleep.
Sit in a comfortable position. Close your eyes, and take a long, slow breath in while tightening one muscle group. When your lungs are completely filled with air, slowly let the breath out as you relax the muscle group. Repeat with different groups of muscles until you have done the whole body.

5. Take a bath

I don't mean to get clean. I am talking about an old fashioned bubble bath. Light candles and even put on some soothing music. Some people even read in the bath. Just soak. If you don't like bubble baths, you could take a mineral bath instead.

6. Shower your stress away

If you are the type who loves a good shower, you can also relieve some of your stress by "washing" it away. You can do this by closing your eyes and taking slow, deep breaths, like the meditation exercise above, but instead of tightening and relaxing muscle groups, imagine the water pulling the stress out of your body as it travels from your head, down your body and into the shower drain. Take your time doing this, concentrating on the water and what it feels like as it travels down your body. The best time to do this exercise is right before you step out of the shower for the night.

Bergamot (Citrus bergamia)

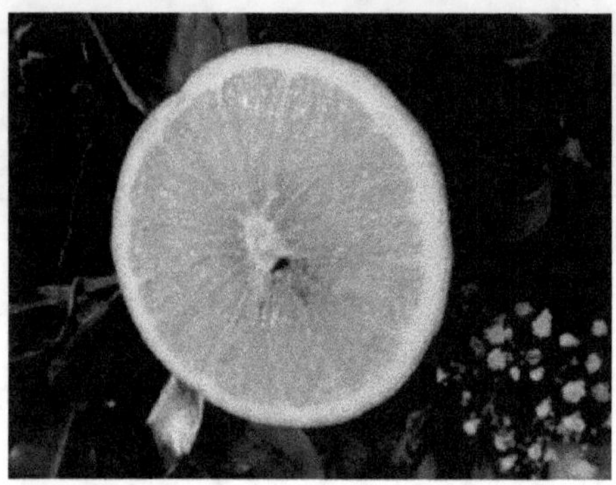

This is an essential oil that is good for calming the nerves, helping relieve depression, and cases of anxiety. It is one of the oils that helps with illnesses tied to stress.

Chamomile, Roman (Chamaemelum)

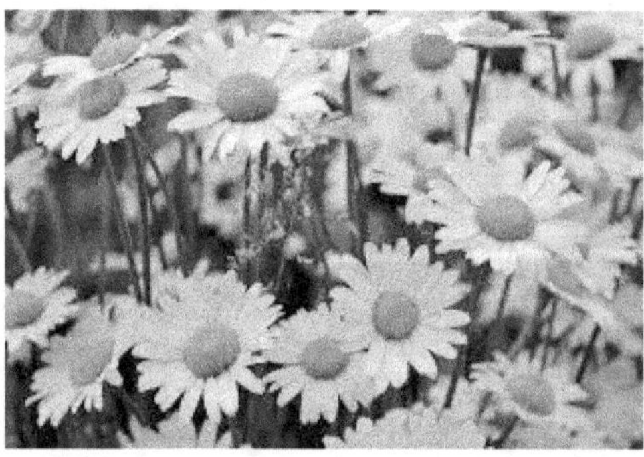

This is a very prevalent essential oil in aromatherapy, and when put in a diffuser blend, it can relieve stress headaches, calm the nerves, and even quell an anxiety attack. It has also been known to alleviate migraines.

Frankincense (Boswellia carteri)

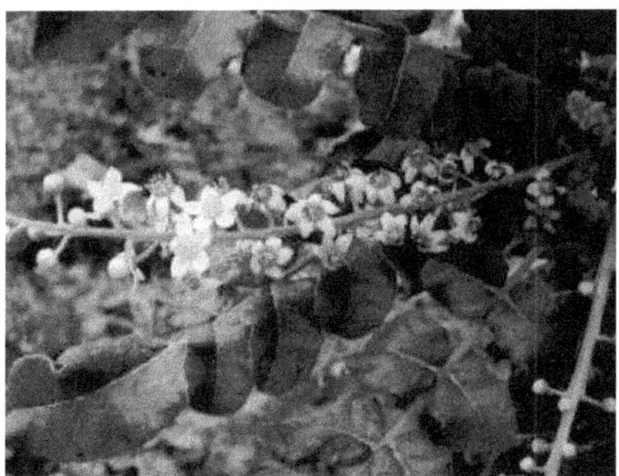

Long used in churches as incense, this essential oil is excellent as soothing frayed nerves due to stress, helps to alleviate anxiety, and also helps to relieve stress-related conditions.

Lavender (Lavandula angustifolia)

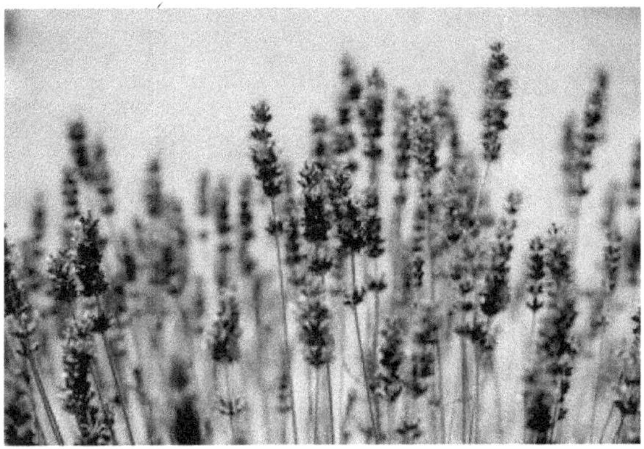

This very versatile essential oil is key in blends when you're wanted to take the stress off of your mind and relax your body. It's also good for helping to treat migraines and stress related headaches.

Rose, Damask (Rosa Damascena)

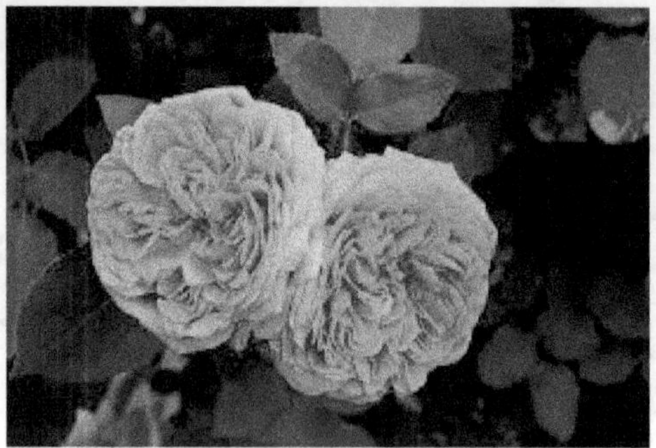

This is one of the more expensive essential oils, but it is very effective in cases of tension headaches, nervous tension, and can help with insomnia.

Vetiver (Vetivera Zizanioides)

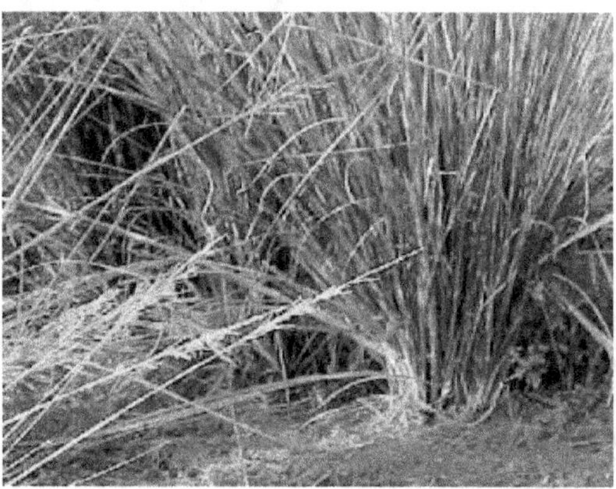

This essential oil has been used to relieve nervous tension, help to induce drowsiness to insomniacs, and has also been used for depression.

Diffuser blends do not need to be diluted. To use them, just mix the oils together in the proportions in the recipes and turn on the diffuser.

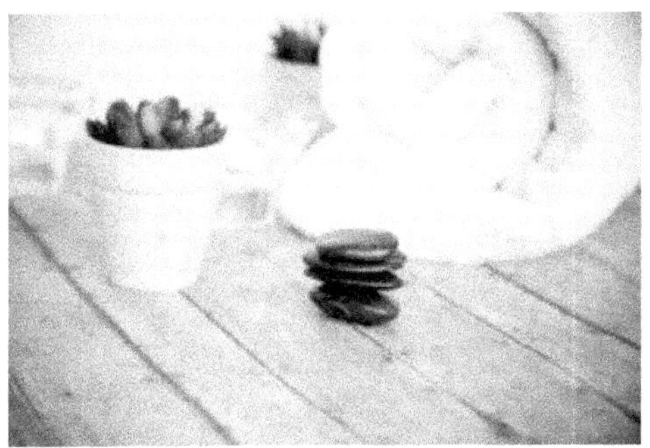

Blend #1

3 Drops Lavender Essential oil

3 Drops Bergamot Essential oil

2 Drops Ylang Ylang

Blend #2

3 Drops of Chamomile Essential oil

3 Drops of Vetiver Essential oil

2 Drops of Frankincense Essential oil

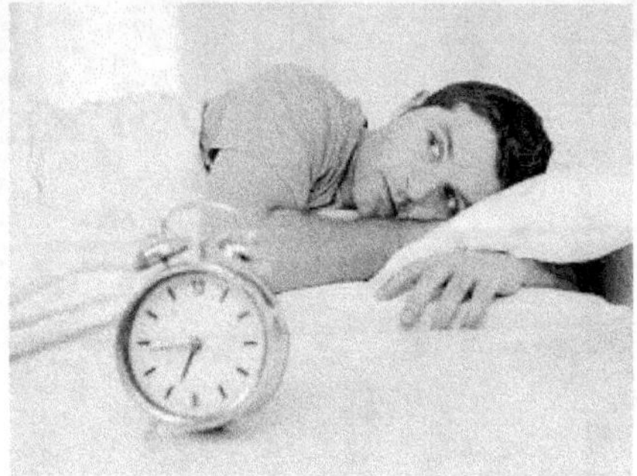

Not being able to sleep can, and often does, cause other mental as well as physical problems. There are many reasons one can suffer from insomnia, but few natural ways to combat it to help you get to sleep and be rejuvenated the next morning.

Essential oils

We've already mentioned Damask Rose and Vetiver, but here are a few more to add to this list:

Cedarwood, Texas (Juniperus ashei)

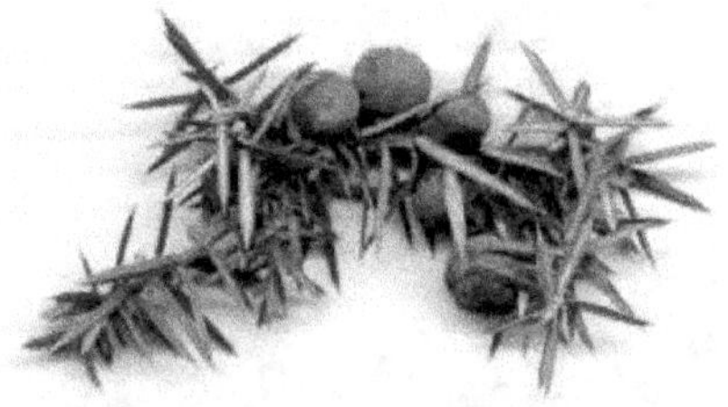

This essential oil brings a mellow wood aroma that can help alleviate stress-related insomnia. This essential oil is quite potent in small amounts and should be avoided if you are pregnant.

Marjoram, Sweet (Origanum marjorana)

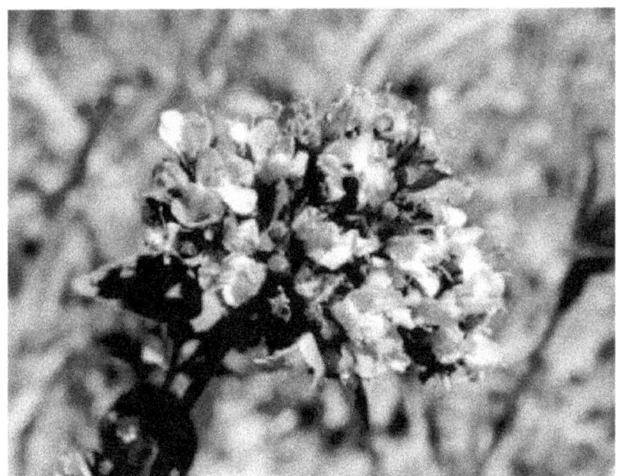

This is an essential oil that is used in many insomnia blends. It's also good for migraines, headaches, and nervous tension. Please, don't use this while pregnant.

Sandalwood (Santalum album)

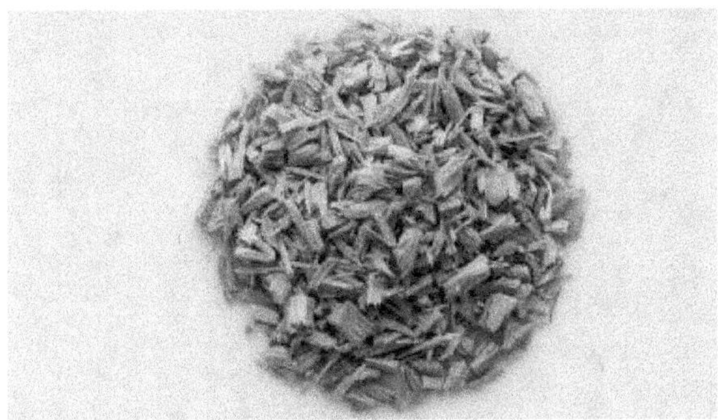

This is another pricey essential oil. It is highly recommended for treating insomnia. It is also very good for elevating mood.

Blend #1

2 Drops Sandalwood Essential oil

2 Drops Marjoram Essential oil

3 Drops Vetiver Essential oil

3 Drops Damask Rose Essential oil

Blend #2

2 Drops Cedarwood Essential oil

2 Drops Sandalwood Essential oil

6 Drops Roman Chamomile Essential oil

Essential oils as Sedatives

Sometimes you just need to relax in order to get to sleep. Your nerves are on edge, and you need to something to calm them.
Among the oils we've already listed,, you can use:

Chamomile
Frankincense
Lavender, and
Marjoram

Here are two more you can add to the list above:

Clary Sage (Salvia sclarea)

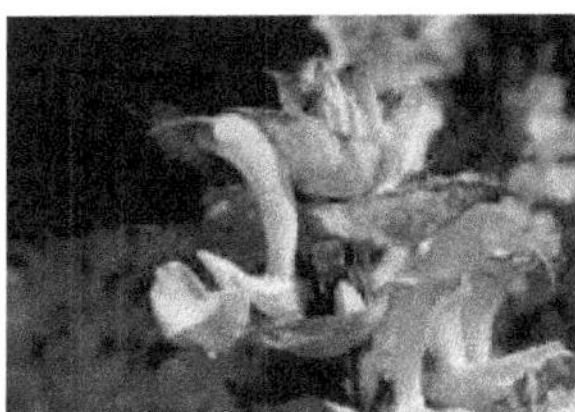

This essential oil is often used to help with depression, migraines, nervous tension, and for stress. Do not use this oil if you are pregnant or drinking. This essential oil is used in small amounts due to its narcotic effect.

Valerian (Valeriana fauriei)

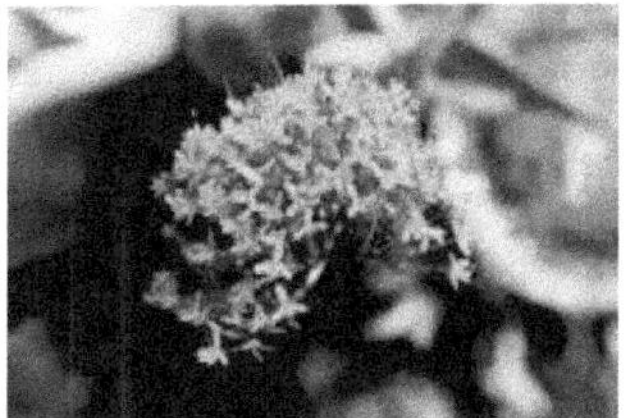

Known as an alternative for Valium, this herb and essential oil calms restlessness, insomnia, and other nervous disorders. Due to the potency of this oil, it is to be used in very small amounts.

Sedative Blend I

1 Drop Valerian Essential oil
2 Drops Clary Sage Essential oil
5 Drops Ylang Ylang Essential oil

Sedative Blend II

2 Drops Valerian Essential oil
4 Drops Cedarwood Essential oil
4 Drops Damask Rose Essential oil

Chapter 3 - Mental Acuity

In this day and age, there are learning disabilities and illnesses that impede our ability to focus on a single task or remembering things from day-to-day.

ADD/ADHD

This is a learning disorder I know all too well. Imagine a web browser in your mind with at least twenty tabs open and all of them are pinging notifications. Your mind is constantly cycling through different thoughts, concepts, and ideas. It can be so debilitating at times you cannot function at all.

Essential oils

Along with essential oils that calm the nerves, those with ADD/ADHD can also use the following essential oils to calm the mind and help you stay focused.
There are many already listed that aid in concentration and calming nervous ticks:
Chamomile, Roman,
Frankincense,
Lavender,
Ylang Ylang, and Vetiver

Here are some to add to the list:

Mandarin (Citrus reticulata)

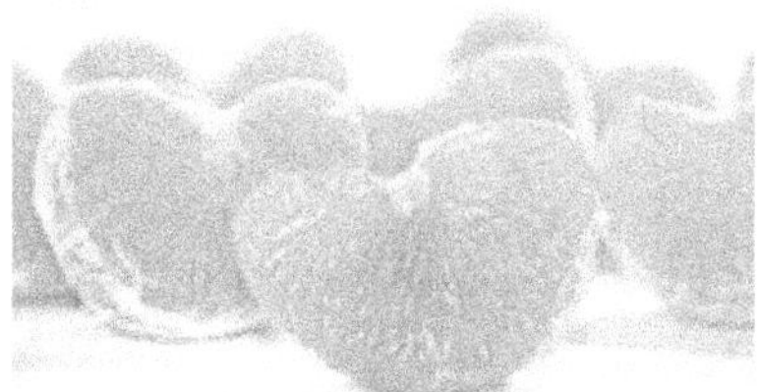

This essential oil is used mainly for children to quiet the mind and help it to focus. It is a mild but effective essential oil.

Patchouli (Pogostemon cablin)

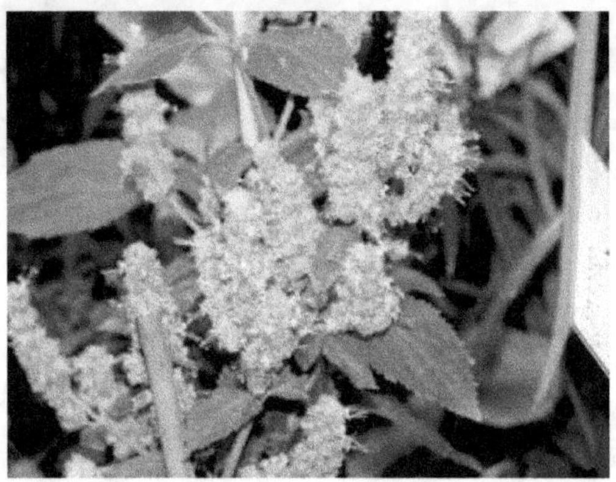

This essential oil is helps to calm the nervous system as a whole which, in turn, helps one to calm the mind and focus.

ADD I

4 Drops Mandarin Essential oil
4 Drops Vetiver Essential oil
2 Drops Frankincense Essential oil

ADD II

4 Drops Patchouli Essential oil
2 Drops Chamomile Essential oil
2 Drops Ylang Ylang Essential oil
2 Drops Clary Sage Essential oil

Memory loss can happen gradually over time. It can also be made worse by senility or dementia. Many of the essential oils in this chapter can be blended with the oils below:

Ginger (Zingiber officinale)

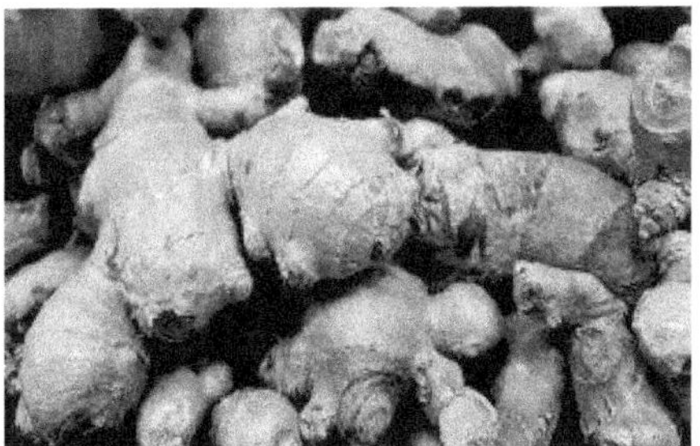

This is a good oil to help correct debilitating mental disorders. It can also boost the action of other essential oils in a blend.

Lemon Balm (Melissa officinalis)

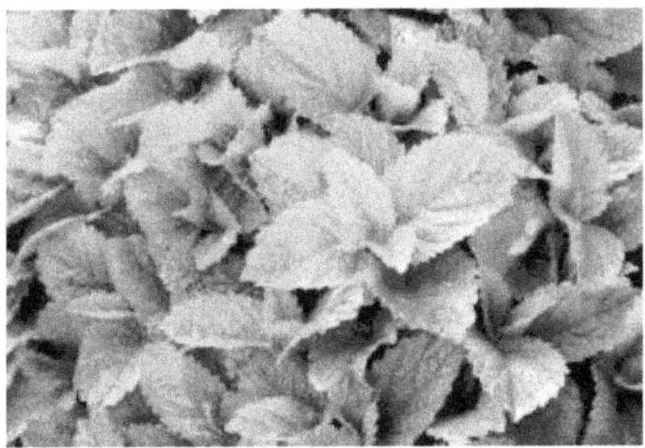

This essential oil helps to clear the fog that is often present in senility and dementia.

Peppermint (Mentha piperita)

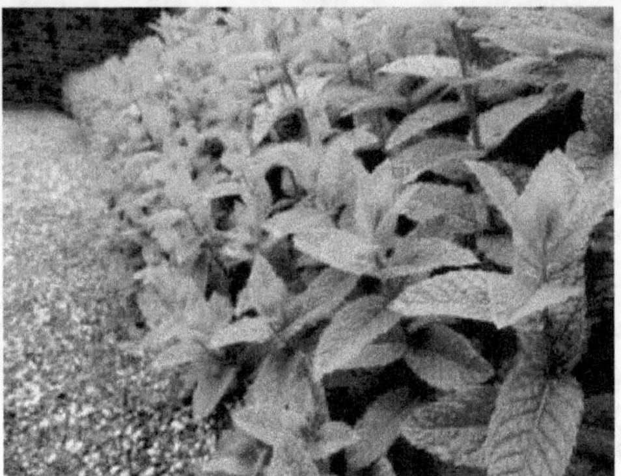

It helps to make the mind more alert and focused. It can also help with clearing migraines and brain fog.

Rosemary (Rosmarinus officinalis)

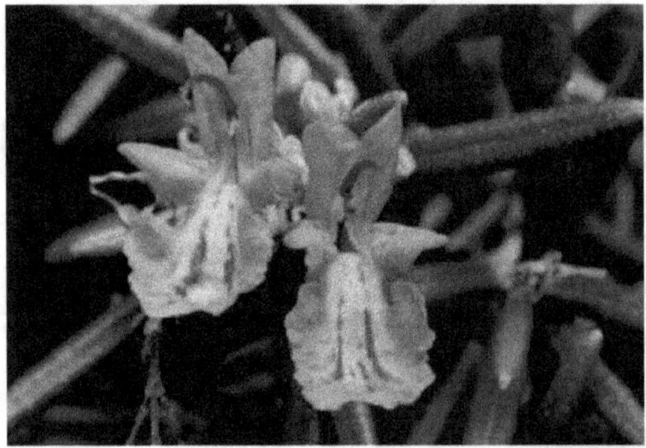

This essential oil and its woody aroma helps with debilitating mental illnesses. It also helps to keep the mind awake and alert. It can trigger epileptic seizures and should be avoided if you have hypertension.

Memory Blend I

4 Drops Lemon Balm Essential oil

4 Drops Peppermint Essential oil

2 Drops Rosemary Essential oil

Memory Blend II

2 Drops Ginger Essential oil

4 Drops Patchouli Essential oil

4 Drops Lemon Balm Essential oil

Knocking Out the Brain Fog

You don't have to have an illness to experience brain fog every now and then. If your groggy, can't seem to focus or just having a hard time getting your mind to perk up so you can get working, that is a type of brain fog, too. You need to knock the cob webs out of there to get your day started and be productive. After, if your brain isn't working at full, neither are you.

Knock out the Cob Webs I

4 Drops Peppermint Essential oil

4 Drops Frankincense

Knock out the Cob Webs II

4 Drops Lemon Essential oil

2 Drops Vetiver Essential oil

2 Drops Peppermint Essential oil

Chapter 4 - In the Bedroom

There are times you wish to be intimate, and I would be remiss if I didn't cover essential oil blends that help keep the spark in the bedroom. There are certain things that can happen when we age to make it difficult to perform. I will cover that as well.

Erectile Dysfunction

For many men, this is the elephant in the room that is too embarrassing to discuss. How does one cope with the inability to perform in the bedroom due to erectile dysfunction. There are many factors that lead to this condition in men, and it's nothing to be ashamed of at all.

1. Stress

Being under stress constantly can lead to a lack of being able to perform. Adding essential oils in a diffuser before you get intimate can help you attain an erection.

2. Dehydration

This may not seem like a big deal and something not often considered, but not having enough fluids in your diet can lead to diminished performance such as starting strong and then your penis going flaccid during sex.

3. Medication

Medications for regulating blood pressure and even some for treating diabetes can lead to erectile dysfunction. One of the best times for optimum performance is to wait until the medication wears off and have intercourse before the next dose is taken.

Clary Sage

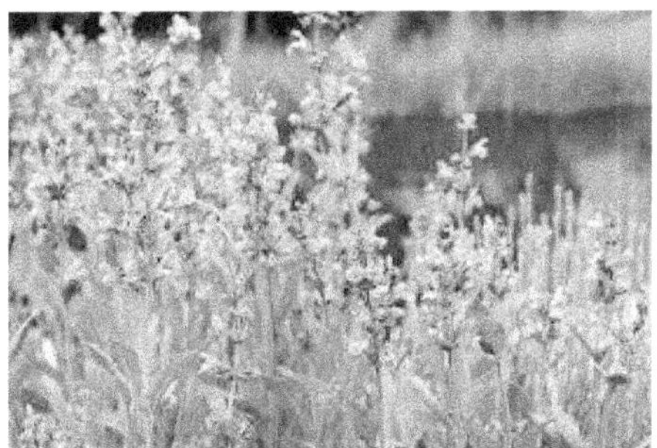

This is a highly recommended oil for impotence. It also helps to increase libido and help with stamina.

Ylang Ylang

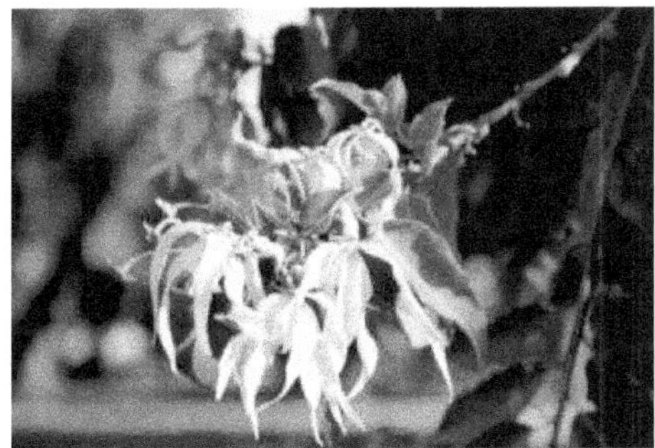

This is good for Erectile dysfunction in that it's calming effects can help attain an erection as well as its euphoric effect.

Peppermint

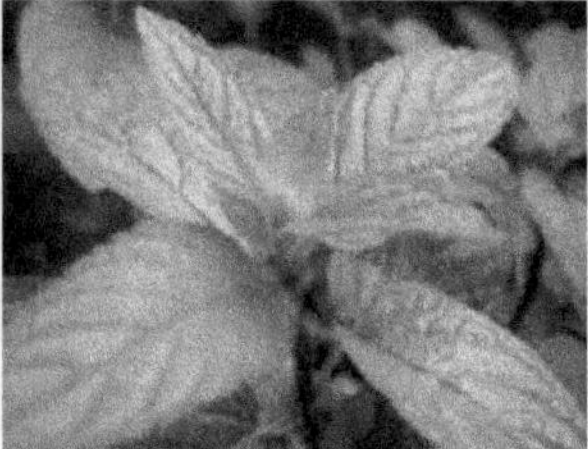

This oil constricts the blood vessels, improving blood pressure and aiding in giving the man an erection.

Cinnamon (Cinnamomum zeylanicum)

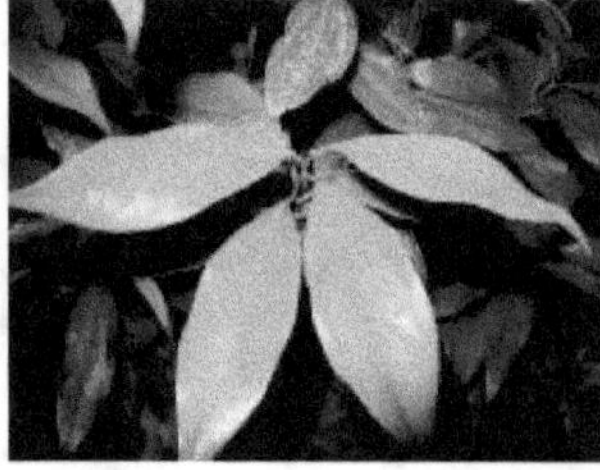

This improves sexual function overall. It is also known to increase libido.

ED Blend I

2 Drops Cinnamon Essential oil
4 Drops Ylang Ylang Essential oil
4 Drops Peppermint Essential oil

ED Blend II

2 Drops Ginger Essential oil
2 Drops Cinnamon Essential oil
4 Drops Lavender Essential oil
4 Drops Rose Essential oil

Clary Sage

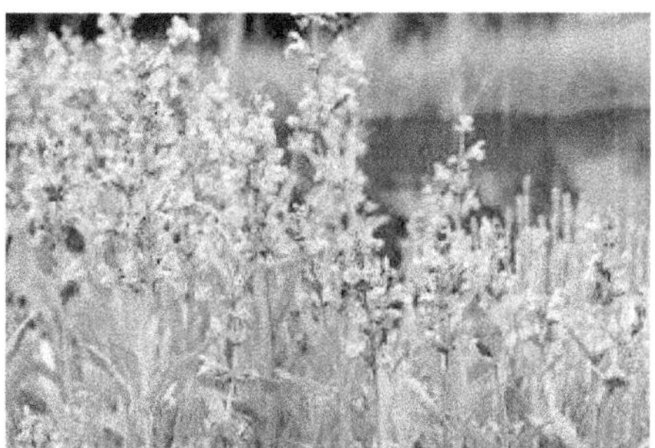

This is a highly recommended oil for impotence. It also helps to increase libido and help with stamina.

Ylang Ylang

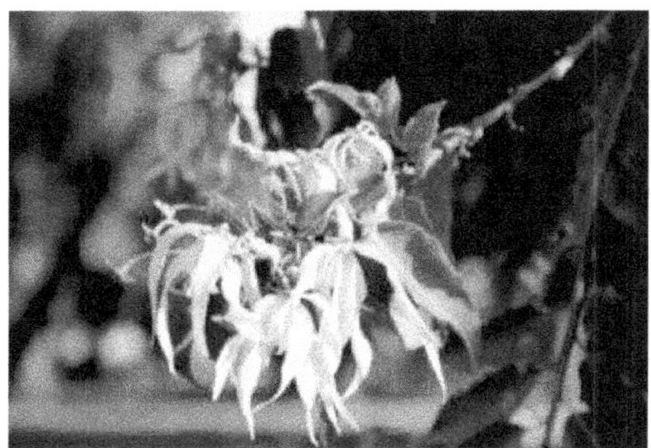

This is good for Erectile dysfunction in that it's calming effects can help attain an erection as well as its euphoric effect.

Peppermint

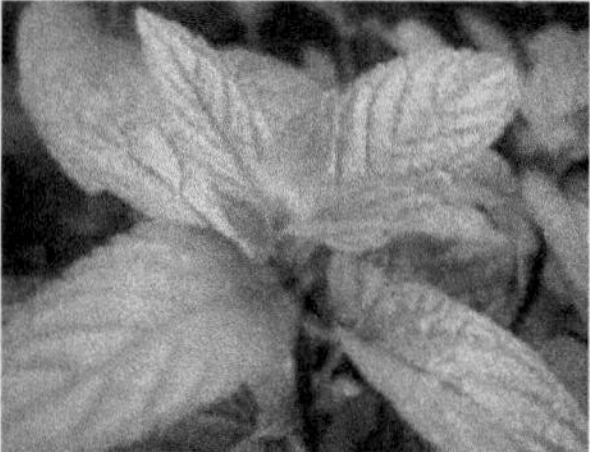

This oil constricts the blood vessels, improving blood pressure and aiding in giving the man an erection.

Cinnamon (Cinnamomum zeylanicum)

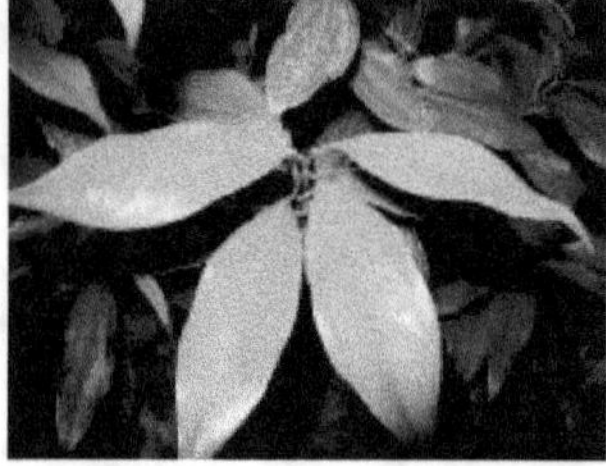

This improves sexual function overall. It is also known to increase libido.

ED Blend I

2 Drops Cinnamon Essential oil

4 Drops Ylang Ylang Essential oil

4 Drops Peppermint Essential oil

ED Blend II

2 Drops Ginger Essential oil

2 Drops Cinnamon Essential oil

4 Drops Lavender Essential oil

4 Drops Rose Essential oil

Low Libido (Low T/Low Estrogen)

Hormone imbalances can cause a lack of desire for sex. This happens naturally as we age. Men have gradual drop in Testosterone as they get older. This, in some cases, can cause a lack of desire.

Decreasing Estrogen levels happen during premenopause and menopause. This too can lead to a lack of interest in sex.

Libido for her I

4 Drops Chamomile Essential oil(natural estrogen)
4 Drops Ylang Ylang Essential oil
2 Drops Cinnamon Essential oil

Libido for her II

4 Drops Jasmine Essential oil (Aphrodisiac for her)
2 Drops Clary Sage Essential oil
2 Drops Black Pepper Essential oil (Sexual Energy)

Libido for him I

4 Drops Damask Rose Essential oil (levels Testosterone)
4 Drops Cardamom Essential oil (Helps with nerves)
2 Drops Black Pepper Essential oil

Libido for him II

4 Drops Ylang Ylang Essential oil
4 Drops Peppermint Essential oil

For him and her I

4 Drops Jasmine Essential oil
4 Drops Ylang Ylang Essential oil

For him and her II

2 Drops Black Pepper Essential oil
4 Drops Peppermint Essential oil
4 Drops Chamomile Essential oil

Chapter 5 - Depression

Depression can take many forms. It can just a case of the blahs to a chemical imbalance to brain which can cause a bi-polar disorder. There are some essential oils which can help lighten the mode and even help even out those bouts of depression. Most of them have already been mentioned. I will provide a few diffuser recipes here.

Helichrysum (Helichrysum angustifolium)

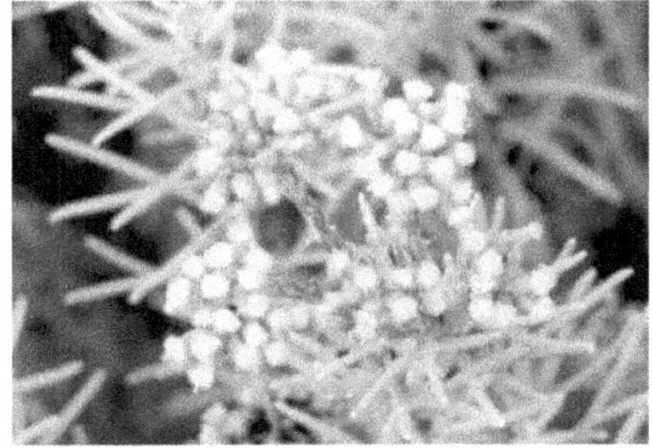

This essential oil may be a bit pricey to some, but it is priceless when it comes to overcoming bouts of depression and the lethargy that comes with it.

Depression Blend I

4 Drops Helichrysum Essential oil

4 Drops Lemon Balm Essential oil

2 Drops Jasmine Essential oil

Depression Blend II

4 Drops Lavender oil

4 Drops Damask Rose Essential oil

2 Drops Bergamot Essential oil

For the Blahs

Sometimes, you just feel off. You have a small case of the mopes and you need a pick-me-up. Here are a couple of recipes you can try to lighten the mood.

Mood Booster I

4 Drops Peppermint Essential oil
2 Drops Orange Blossom Essential oil
2 Drops Ginger Essential oil

Mood Booster II

4 Drops Chamomile Essential oil
2 Drops Ylang Ylang Essential oil
2 Drops Sandalwood Essential oil

Chapter 6 - Children

When fixing essential oil blends for children, you have to keep in not all essential oils can be good for them depending on their age. I will focus on essential oils that are safe for children from twelve months up. Here is a list of some already mentioned: Chamomile, Roman, Lavender, and Peppermint.

Essential oils

Geranium (Pelargonium graveolens)

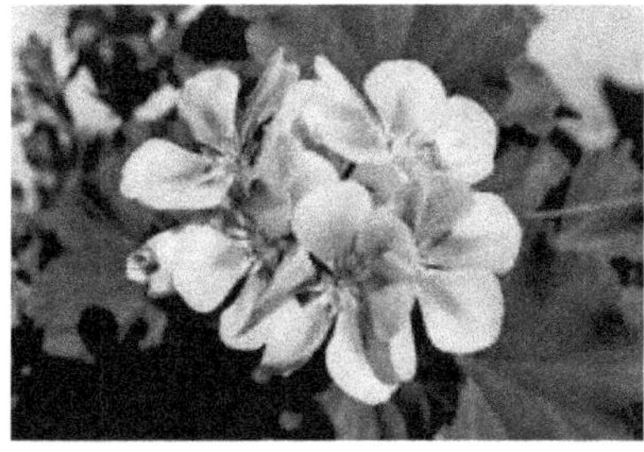

This essential oil is very useful when calming children that are either hyper-active or all still energetic from playing outside.

Palma rosa (Cymbopgon martinii)

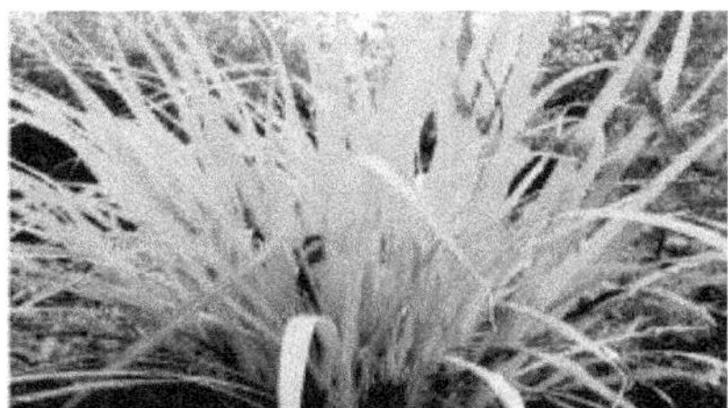

This oil can help with mental exhaustion in children, helping them focus better.

Homework Blend

2 Drops Peppermint Essential oil
2 Drops Palma rosa
2 Drops Geranium (calms nerves/brings down energy levels)

Homework Blend II

4 Drops Lavender Essential oil
4 Drops Peppermint Essential oil

Bed Time I

2 Drops Lavender Essential oil
2 Drops Geranium Essential oil

Bed Time II

3 Drops Palma rosa Essential oil
2 Drops Chamomile Essential oil

Hyper Blend I

4 Drops Peppermint Essential oil
2 Drops Lavender Essential oil

Hyper Blend II

2 Drops Chamomile Essential oil
3 Drops Mandarin Essential oil

Chapter 7 - Blending and other Advice

You can't talk about aromatherapy and essential oils without giving advice on how to make your own, how to store them, and how to care for your oils.

Blending Your Own Recipes

Take the time to smell the individual essential oils before making the blends. It's a good idea to take notes on how each one affects you. This is the best way to make blends tailored specifically to you. Even though I did list what to expect from each essential oil, they can still differ from person to person depending on metabolism.

Notes

Each essential oil has a note or properties that dictate how long it will last.

Top notes

These are lightly scented essential oils which tend to last for about thirty minutes. This are generally citrus oils and mint oils.

Middle Notes

These are evenly scented notes that tend to last for an hour or two. Generally these are normally floral scents.

Bottom Notes

These are heavier, more musky notes and tend to be your tree bark, resin, and more herbal essential oils. These tend to last for up to four hours.

Blending

Since the bottom notes last the longest, you don't to use as much of these. This is fortunate due to the fact many of these types of essential oils tend to be pricey.

Here is an example:

4 Drops Peppermint
3 Drops Lavender
2 Drops Frankincense

The bottom notes also tend to be an anchor to the lighter notes, making them last longer in the blend over all. This is called synergy. A blend that has good synergy will also have more potent effects.

Storage and shelf life

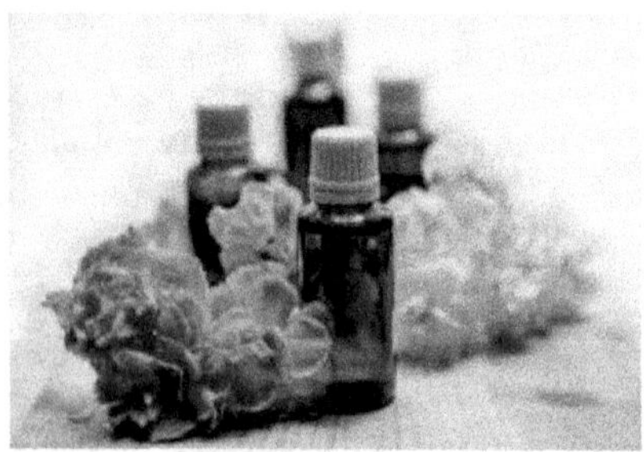

Most of these recipes are to be used after you blend them, but if you want to make enough to store so you have to blend them every time you want to use them, make sure you store them in a cool dark place.

Essential oils, when stored this way, keep their max potency for up to two years. This doesn't mean they don't work at all after the two year period, just that they aren't as strong.

Keep out of Reach

Keep any and all essential oils and blends out of the reach of children and pets. They can have toxic effects.

Do not use without diluting

Never use undiluted essential oils on your skin or in other products like bath salts. You will have to mix them with carrier oils. Undiluted essential oils can cause contact dermatitis. This means it can make your skin break out in a rash or welts due to contact.

Wear Gloves

It is best to always wear gloves when mixing essential oils to make sure they don't come in direct contact with your skin.

Read the label/Research

When buying essential oils, it is important that you know what to expect from those oils. There is plenty of information online, but the best websites are the ones who have been around for a long time and have dedicated their site to the uses essential oils in aromatherapy. DoTerra is not one I would recommend for information. Aromaweb is excellent and can provide you with a wealth of information on essential oils and aromatherapy as whole should you wish to expand your interest in essential oils.

Join Forums

There are many forums and online groups that help you with advice, blending, and uses of essential oils. Many of the people in these forums are kind, helpful, and some are even licensed in aromatherapy.

Branch out

With over 90 different essentials, there is no need to stop with the ones in this book. You can use oils for first aid, digestion, and a myriad of other uses. You may find you like using certain oils more than others.

Experiment

Make your own diffuser blends and see if they work better for you than the ones in this book. These are just meant to get you started.

Use them to boost lotions

You can add up to six drops of essential oils to one tablespoon of lotion to boost the lotion's effects. You can turn a simple moisturizer into a treatment for a sunburn, to treat bad rashes, and even to help your skin when you add them to your nightly facial routine.

Conclusion

This is virtually no end to the ways you can use essential oils. Just make sure you are using them in the way they were intended. Essential oils can enrich every part of your life and improve your well-being. Keep an ear to the ground, so to speak. There are new discoveries every year, and every year people are finding more and more uses for essential oils in their lives.

Aromatherapy is a wonderful way to take charge of your health and can open doors to other types of holistic healing. It is a time-honored natural health field which has gained popularity in the last decade or so. There is always something new to learn.

I hope this book has helped you in your quest for knowledge on essential oils and their uses. Be on the look-out for more books in this series. Never stop learning. Never stop taking charge of your health.